10 Years On

Book 7 in the surviving a
Stroke Series

By

Dr Andy Hill

Contents

Dedication

To Stroke Survivors everywhere

and to their carers

and all NHS staff, you are the best in the world!

Introduction

On Saturday 5th November 2010, rather unusually developing throughout the day, I suffered a significant Right Anterior Ischaemic Stroke.

This book continues the story of the after-effects of this Stroke and the fact that I was one of the middle group of stroke patients, those who survive but with life-changing after-effects.

I will try to explain the somehow indescribable, many-faceted effects of a stroke.

How they develop, change and continue 10 Years On.

[The non-medical]

Dr Andy Hill.

Physical Effects

Initially, I was left with a total paralysis of my left arm and leg.

During the first week in the hospital, not content with having had a stroke, I suffered a non-occluded DVT, a clot in a major vein of my left leg, my Stroke affected side, as well as a small pulmonary embolism at the base of my right lung.

The DVT was incredibly painful. I was immediately put on Clexane followed by a six-month course of Warfarin. No further problems were caused by the DVT or Pulmonary Embolism, although Warfarin caused several minor bleeding problems and the frequent visits to the Anticoagulant Clinic were a little tiresome.

After the six months of Warfarin, I was moved on to daily doses of Clopidogrel, for the foreseeable future. This is the standard Antiplatelet treatment following a stroke.

The DVT caused a weeks delay in the start of my physiotherapy.

But thee time I left the hospital after seven weeks I was able to walk a few steps with the aid of a stick but also had an electric wheelchair for use indoors and a small wheel, non-self-propelling wheelchair for use outdoors.

Physiotherapy continued, at home for six weeks and then as a hospital outpatient for about one year.

At the end of this period, I could walk proficiently with a stick for short distances and had some rudimentary, useful movement of my left arm.

Over the next few years, my walking improved, as did the movement in my arm, amazingly driving helped improvement, even though I had an automatic gearbox car with adaptations to make it operable with my right hand only. I soon found that I was using my left hand more and more, which increases available movement further.

Unfortunately, after about four years, I started to experience both acute and chronic pain in my hips, especially the left, my stroke side.

After a short period of diagnosis and x-rays, I was diagnosed with early-stage Osteoarthritis in both hips.

As a result, my mobility started to decline again. A couple of years later, I started having problems with my left knee. It was assumed but never fully diagnosed that this too was early-stage Osteoarthritis. I underwent a couple of short courses of physiotherapy, which gave me a set of physio exercises to do daily to halt the deterioration and keep the mobility of the joints.

I now live with a balance of doing just the right level and type of exercise, to maintain some level of fitness and mobility against the pain, both acute and chronic that arthritis gives me.

I addition to the joint pain, I also have a level of neuropathic pain.

My pain is currently managed by maximum dose paracetamol, 20mg Amitriptyline and Morphine, administered as Codeine Phosphate and prolonged release Morphine Sulfate, with a Morphine equivalent dose of between 39mg and 69mg per day.

This physiotherapy and analgesic routine is pretty much wholly effective, apart from the occasional moderate to severe acute episodes, caused by the wrong type of movement or exercise. I am particularly prone to acute pain caused by prolonged standing or sitting.

Arthritis and pain aside, my mobility is stable and acceptable now, although I am classified as severely disabled, unable to walk more than 20m without pain.

Mental / Psychological Effects

Before I had my Stroke, what little I knew about them was limited just to the physical effects. However, I suppose that anything that involves an injury to the brain is bound to cause some mental effects.

As it happened, I quickly realised that the Stroke was having a profound effect on my thinking.

As I was settling down to my first night in hospital, I decided I wanted to get to sleep. So I turned to a simple breathing exercise that I knew, simply following your breath patterns with "The breath flows in", "The breath flows out". After a while, I would change it to simply "In", "Out", on this occasion I never got out of the longer version, and I was asleep.

I woke around 6 am thinking "Great, I'm still alive!" The ward was starting to wake up, nurses rounds, Obs, Drugs. A routine I would get used to over the next seven weeks.

My thinking was indeed messed up, especially in the first couple of weeks.

Some of the events that illustrated this, although I didn't realise it at the time were:-

Confusion over room layout.

For the first week, I was in a side room, which had the entrance from the ward at the far end of the wall to the left of my bed, also the entrance to the toilet at the extreme right end of the wall opposite my bed.

Because at this time, the entire left side of my body was paralysed, I never visited this toilet, I used urinal bottles and was hoisted onto a bedpan.

One evening I got confused between the doors and wondered why people kept coming in and out of my toilet.

End of the world scenario.

While watching TV one evening, I started to feel tired, so I pushed the TV, which was mounted on a moveable arm, up and away from my bed.

I must have been watching some "Everyone in the world has died film or documentary discussion".

The TV was still on, with the sound still audible and I drifted off to sleep. The sound from the TV merged into a dream. Then the program must have ended and moved on to the news or something, anyway I awoke, and from the ward, I could hear here nurse call bleepers going off in various places and wondered why aren't they getting answered? I then began to think I was the only person left alive.

I was really relieved when a nurse came in and asked if she could turn off the TV.

The everyone is against me paranoia.

In the other side room just across a corridor from mine, was a lady named Doris, who would chat incessantly to the nurses when they were tending to her and to herself when she was alone.

I was a frequent user of the buzzer at this time due to confusion, and regular real or perceived needs. One day I buzzed my buzzer when there was a nurse in with Doris, who then said: "I'll have to go, Andy, is buzzing." Every time I used the buzzer after this, or even when she heard someone else's buzzer, she would say "Andy is buzzing again".

Then one day when I was dozing or otherwise incredibly confused, I could hear Doris talking about me and saying something about, "He's evil, you know". For some time after this, I became paranoid every time I could hear her talking, worried she was going to report me to the staff or something.

Word and phrase analysis.

I would frequently latch on to particular words I heard or thought of.

One day I heard the Name Sheila mentioned and thought "Sheila, S h e I l a, unless it's the Irish spelling, Sheighla, no Sheiaghla no ...", this seemed to go round in my head for ages.

On another occasion I heard a nurse say to someone else, "I'm just going to get Doris' Diamorphine from the safe, can you...". I then thought "Diamorphine, that's Heroin.". Then this thought went round my mind for what seemed like ages.

All of the above happened in my first week in the hospital, a crazy week indeed!

A week or so later, when I had been moved to the central part of the ward after contracting a nasty urinary tract infection. I had a sort of epiphany, in which I realised that I had, kind of, started a new life, and everything that had happened up until now was irrelevant, and life was all about moving forward.

Then the idea kept, repeating in my mind, "Everything up until now is irrelevant, no everything up until NOW, no NOW………" etc. until I thought "As long as I don't go out and kill anyone!"

I also had many dreams that blended into reality, during that hazy time of being half asleep and half awake.

This was an extension of the "End of world scenario" mentioned above; an example of this was.

Networking the obs machines.

Every morning when on the main part of the word, it was usual to be woken up by the beeping of obs machines as nurses came round checking blood pressure, and other observations.

One morning I was half asleep, and the beeping of the machines found their way into my dream, and I was discussing with IT colleges how to network the obs machines and automate the updating of patient records.

A note on depression

Writing of this book had stalled for several weeks. I had lost my muse.

As will be discussed shortly, Once I left the hospital, I started suffering post-stroke anxiety, which was initially severely acute.

During the diagnosis and early treatment of this, I discovered that I was also suffering from depression but didn't realise this.

I believe that it is depression that triggered this writing lapse, causing a loss of motivation and energy.

I decided that sharing this would provide the impetus to start writing again.

It has!

End note

The confusion was worst during the first two weeks, post-stroke gradually reducing as the weeks past. Once this had happened, the motivation to recover and get home began to grow. I made a lot of effort in both Physio and Occupational therapy.

When asked when I was looking to be discharged, I said I wanted to be home for Christmas (I was admitted on 6th November). The therapy was then focussed on working towards this.

I was finally discharged on 20th December, and so began the next phase of my recovery.

I was taken home by ambulance, my parents, who lived just across the road, were there to meet me. They stayed for a while and then left although my mother had decided she was going to spend the nights in my spare room. I expected this and didn't argue.

Once they had left, I felt so alone, didn't know what to do with myself.

However, I soon settled into a routine, mother staying at night, my father also visiting in the evenings. I also had carers visiting three times a day and therapists every few days. I also had to attend Warfarin Clinic initially weekly then two weekly then monthly for six months following my DVT.

I couldn't settle, terrible anxiety set in. I was afraid and worried about everything.

The therapists taught me relaxation techniques which helped a bit. Still, occasionally I would get terrible anxiety attacks from time to time which would even present physical symptoms, on two occasions during the first three months, I ended up attending A&E with chest pains.

Strangely fear of another Stroke didn't cause these attacks but just about anything else did, including anxiety about the anxiety.

One morning I woke up with some minor pain or other, thinking " Oh what now, it's nothing serious, but what if it is, why do I keep getting this anxiety? Well if it is something serious and I die, at least I'll be rid of this anguish. NO!

This thought was enough to spur me into action, I called the Stroke Matron, and she came to visit me later that day.

I talked her through what was happening, and she told me that I needed to go on SSRI anti-depressants. This was a surprise to me, I was expecting some counselling, but she said to me that post-stroke your serotonin levels drop, for reasons that are not well understood.

So I duly made an appointment to see my Doctor and was put on a repeat prescription of Sertraline 50mg per day.

So began a new chapter.

The stroke matron warned me that the anxiety would initially get worse on the medication, but after two weeks, it would settle down, and I would feel the relieving effect of the medication. This was the understatement of all time, the anxiety increased noticeably, and I seemed to have every side effect mentioned on the patient information leaflet, except for the severe ones.

However, I convinced myself that it would all pass and I would feel better. Sure enough, after about two weeks during my daily visit to my parents, I suddenly realised that the anxiety and gone and that I felt alive again.

I bathed in the glory of being anxiety-free for maybe a few weeks. Then out of the blue something happened to make me feel anxious again, initially, I thought that my respite was over, but thankfully I quickly realised that, yes I was feeling anxious, but I realised that it was just anxiety and I was able to stop it spiralling out of control.

As time has gone on, I have realised that the anxiety is still there under the surface, but I can control it. Admittedly I sometimes manage the anxiety by removing myself from the anxiety-causing situation. However removing yourself from the situation, is a valid coping strategy.

A few months later, at another doctor's appointment, I was explaining that the anxiety was still there and asked if we should increase the medication dose? His response was that before increasing the dose, I should try counselling. I agreed to this, and at my preliminary session I was told that my coping strategies were sufficient and if I continued on the current dose of medication unless I found that I felt I needed a higher dose and this would be her recommendation to my GP.

This point of view changed my perspective a little and weighing up the increased side effects of a higher dose with how I now felt. I decided to maintain my current dose and concentrate on my coping strategies to manage the residual anxiety. To date, this has continued to work well.

Initially, I feared that they would take me off the medication at some point. My response to this would be unless they could guarantee that I wouldn't feel like I had before starting the medication, then I didn't want to come off it.

I brought this view up in a few reviews over the years, and so far, I remain on the medication. I have also managed to build up around a year's supply to avoid any possible interruption of the dose, which is very important for anti-depressants.

Memory.

Immediately after my Stroke, I found my short term and working (very short term) memories took a hit.

I had learnt that this was expected following a stroke, so I was not overly concerned.

However, a few years later, I noticed that my short term and working memories had started to deteriorate again, so I consulted with the Doctor again. At this point, I discovered that one of the first checks for memory deterioration is to test for anxiety and/or depression. The tests for these took the form of a questionnaire, which I took away to complete, I also had a series of blood tests, at my next appointment the questionnaire indicated that anxiety/depression was not the issue and the blood test indicated that there was no chemical cause.

I was referred to the mental health team, who visited me at home and took me through a series of tests. The outcome of this was that I was mentally sound but with some deficiencies in the short term and working memory, vocabulary and fluency. The consultant decided that there was no need for further action at this point, but I should monitor it and get a further referral if I noticed any other significant deterioration.

To date, I have not.

Changes to ambitions and life goals

At the time of my Stroke, I had just started what was expected to be the final year of my PhD research project.

I planned to use my PhD to move on from what I considered to be a dead-end job in a small company.

My first thought was that this was all over now. The first few months post-stroke did not provide any encouragement either, as I had quickly realised that my ability to hold down a full-time job as lost.

However, thankfully, as the PhD research was a joint project, with my research partner having already secured a job in Germany, on the basis that she was working on her PhD. One of the proposed possibilities was that I would join her over there.

As it happened my research partner, was petitioning the university, that as the research was now in the conclusion and documentation and I had already contributed significantly to what was always mean to be a shared thesis. All of this was going on unbeknownst to me to not falsely build up my hopes.

The university was happy with this and six months after my partner graduated, I was also awarded my PhD. I missed out on the awards ceremony, though.

Unfortunately due to my post-stroke problems, apart from calling myself Dr. and a bit of remote consultancy for my research partners company in Germany, I have not so far done a lot with my PhD.

However, I still consider it quite an achievement.

Conclusions

So, what have I learnt in the ten years following my Stroke?

Well, life certainly changed with the Stroke but not all in a negative way.

Before I had my Stroke, I knew little about it, but thanks to the FAST campaign, I knew how to recognise one.

In the morning, when the first signs appeared, a strange numbness in my left hand, I immediately performed the FAST test on myself. Raised my arms above my head, checked my facial symmetry in the mirror and spoke out loud to check my speech wasn't slurred, at this point I passed OK.

Later in the afternoon at my parents, when I couldn't get up from the sofa and my left side became paralysed and my speech slurred, I knew exactly what was happening. I also remembered that strokes could cause unconsciousness and seizures, I figured that as I wasn't having either of these, I just thought I was doing well.

During my time in the hospital, I had a kind of epiphany, and this was along the lines of, everything that had happened up until now didn't matter now, what mattered was to move forward making the most of what I had. I saw it as starting a new life, a different life, but as valid and vital as my old life.

The early days out of the hospital were difficult, mainly before I got the anxiety under control.

I quickly realised I wouldn't be able to go back to work as before, I didn't have the energy or stamina, and as it turned out, the company didn't want me back anyway.

Some people would say this is a defeatist attitude, but I found it essential that I should enjoy my new life, and it not be a chore.

Having said this, I firmly believe that you have to take little excursions outside your comfort zone to challenge yourself and allow yourself to move forward occasionally. However, these excursions shouldn't be so far that you fail and get disheartened.

Recovering from a stroke is a long game. My consultant described it like trying to eat an elephant. You have to do it in small pieces.

It is sometimes said that any function you have not recovered within six months of a stroke, you will never recover. I know this not to be true. Recovery indeed is quickest within the first six months, but small stage recovery continues for years afterwards.

For example, it took almost a year for me to get any useful recovery of movement in my Stroke affected arm and improvements are continuing today.

I will repeat those things you were good at before your Stroke recover much quicker than things you were not so good at, essential things tend to recover quicker than mere nice to have things. Your brain subconsciously prioritises these things.

Most importantly, you need to want to recover but at the same time, learn to live within the restrictions that you have at any one time.

As with everything, a positive mental attitude is critical, concentrate on the positive, the things that you can do, rather than the things you cannot do, yet!

Positive support from family and friends is necessary too. It's no good having an excellent positive attitude yourself if you then allow those around you to drag you down.

Within the first year of my recovery, I was visited by a fellow stroke survivor, a practice which is encouraged to allow people who know what each other are going through, to offer mutual support.

In his first visit, he was quite down about his recovery, so I told him about a positive attitude, and he seemed to welcome the idea. The next time I saw him, he was much more optimistic about his recovery but somewhat dismissive of mine. I found this negativity disappointing. We didn't see each other much after that.

Not all stroke survivors are a "good fit" for supporting each other, as with all relationships in life, you have to pick your partners carefully.

Finally, I know that this is common amongst stroke survivors, but I seem to be significantly affected by it. I have developed an intolerance to people who moan and waste time not getting to the point. I'm not sure if this is due to knowing how precious life is or because I think people's inconveniences are nothing compared to what I have to put up with.

I have an almost autistic trait of not being able to cope with things that do not go exactly to plan and people who don't listen to me.

The final word is to try to avoid having a stroke by living a healthy lifestyle, don't smoke, drink excessively, eat too much salt, keep your weight down.

If you are unlucky enough to have a stroke but lucky enough to be one of the 2/3s that survive. Improve your lifestyle as mentioned above, be positive, strive for gradual improvements, keep going, appreciate that life will be different and learn to embrace your new lifestyle, life is still better than the alternative.

If you know someone who has had a stroke, be positive with them and for them. Listen to them, as with all disabilities, don't fly at them thinking you can help, ask them if you can help a follow what they say!

It's ten years on and the time seems to have flown, I am a born again stroke survivor, I embrace my new life, I am happy. However, my mantra remains,

Don't have a Stroke; they're Rubbish!

End Note

This book was written during the great COVID-19 pandemic of 2020.

For the same reasons that flu causes a greater risk in stroke survivors, I believed that the COVID infection posed the same risks to me, although at the time opinion was divided on this.

Although the Stroke Association were funding research into such links.